Essential Oils for Colds

Essential Oil Recipes for
Colds
for Diffusers, Roller Bottles,
Inhalers & more.

Rica V. Gadi

Printed in the United States of America

First Printing, 2019

ISBN: 9781086035568

http://eorecipes.net

This book is dedicated to all the strong people who are taking responsibility for your own well being and doing something to be better.

All my heartfelt gratitude to the following people: my mom Ruby Jane, you have made me everything I am today; my dad Nestor-- my eternal, my angel, and the source of my perseverance; Mommyling, my spiritual guide ; Ria & Joe, the true witnesses of my transformation and my foundation pillars; Ellie Jane, the sparkle of our eyes;

Juan, thanks for always encouraging me to push harder - you are my ONE; Rocco & Radha, my reason for everything.

The Love of my family and friends is the fountain of inspiration that never runs dry. Thank you for constantly inspiring me, motivating me, and loving me unconditionally.

This book will never be complete without the help of my trusted and talented friends the #NOWsuperstars and my #oilbularya friends

Blending Essential Oils to use for a very specific reason has become very popular in recent years. There are several reasons why this is so. Blending EOs is basically about inhaling - as it has been proven that aromas have the ability to trigger feelings, emotions and personal memories.

With this in mind, it is obvious that everyone is unique when it comes to what triggers your senses. It all boils down to personal preference for the aroma to trigger what you want to unleash. Everyone is different and we all connect to the aroma differently, so what might work for one might not work for another person.

Of course, we also want the blend we personalize to be therapeutic. This is the best reason why to blend essential oils. We want the blend we create to help us with a very specific emotion or physical condition. As much as smelling good is important in a blend, it is more important that we blend oils that are not only pleasing to the smell but also produces the therapeutic effect we are after.

Then you have to think about contraindications. Making sure the blend you create is safe to use.

I suggest that before blending find out if the oils you are using is safe for a condition you may have example, if you are pregnant, or have specific allergies. Consult your physician prior to moving forward.

The recipes I have in this book is a compilation of what has proven to work and favored by hundreds of EO enthusiasts. It takes out the guesswork to get you started.

Again, we urge you to read the recipes and make sure that this is safe for you to try.

The book is very specific to a physical and emotional condition. There are several recipes here because you might want to rotate and you may like one and not the other. There is also a variety of applications. Some of us prefer to diffuse, some to make roller bottles, and others to create inhalers and sprays.

I hope you enjoy this compilation, feel free to use the notes section and jot down your fave blends. There is a wonderful world of EO blending - this is just the beginning.

Rica

The most familiar viral infection that almost every person has encountered in their life is having a common cold. As the name suggests, it is very common because it can result from the more than 200 types of viruses. Even researchers are not yet certain of the real number of viruses available that everyone can be exposed to. A common cold is usually caught from individuals that already have the virus or it may be from exposure to cold germs and other contaminated objects. It is fairly easy to catch and may enter from the mouth, nose or eyes, but it is not very dangerous as long as it is treated properly.

Common colds are usually associated with symptoms like a runny nose and congestion, coughing and sore throat. Oftentimes common colds also go hand in hand with the flu. It is common to experience additional symptoms such as a headache, fever and muscle pain whenever a cold is paired with the flu. These symptoms usually last for only 10 days or less. Over-the-counter medicines can be used to treat the common cold and it is usually not severely dangerous for your health. Most people claim that having colds are actually a good thing as the body discovers new viruses and adopts immunity over it during the course of infection.

There are several remedies for colds from over-the-counter medication to taking vitamins, lozenges and eating warm food like soups. A natural remedy that is becoming more popular to many people because of its versatility and effectiveness is the use of essential oils. They are plant extracts that have many different properties that can help in different problem areas of the body. Essential oils are a great natural alternative to remedy colds and flu. Some regularly use it to prevent any form of infections in general because these oils are known for their antibacterial properties.

There are many ways to use essential oils to help with pain and just overall relief for symptoms like headaches, muscle sores, and congestions. Essential oils can be inhaled from a diffuser, which is best used for symptoms like sinus. It can also be diluted with a carrier oil to apply topically to soothe muscle sores and tensions. Oregano is a much recommended essential oil that a lot of herbalists use because of its antiviral and antibacterial benefits. It is one of the best plants to fight bacteria and also helps soothe inflammation. Other oils such as lime, thyme, and eucalyptus also have antiseptic and soothing properties good to fight against symptoms like coughs and sore throats.

Table of Contents

Best Essential Oils for Colds

Due to climate change, there are also changes in the weather patterns. These changes cause bad health conditions due to the adaptability of our body. To be specific, it primarily affects our respiratory system especially if our immune system is not boosted. Common example of the sickness we get from climate change is colds. Let us all admit that cough are pretty much irritating and give us discomfort wherever we are. This ailment also disrupts us from our slumber for some instances. Everyone has different ways of medication, may it be through prescribed medicines or herbal medicines. However, with modern medicine, researchers utilized the technology to develop natural treatment, the rise of essential oils. There are a plethora of essential oils in the market, but since we aim to help individuals who suffer from respiratory ailments, we listed some of the most recommended essential oils for colds.

- Eucalyptus
  We can't deny the fact that eucalyptus oil is recognized for its ability to treat respiratory ailments such as cough. It helps you clean the microorganisms and toxins in your body as it acts as an expectorant. It also helps you fight the bacteria that cause your cough and cold

since it has an antimicrobial effect. Eucalyptus may also help relieve muscle pain and tension, and inflammation resulting from cold, cough, or flu.
For inhalation process, add 10-15 drops of eucalyptus essential oil to a bowl of boiling water. Just simply breathe in the vaporized soothing scent for at least 5-10 minutes while it tries to calm and clear your nasal cavity. You may also try to mix a drop of eucalyptus oil and 3 drops of lavender oil in a cup of hot water, dampen a washcloth in the mixture and directly apply to your forehead as the lavender oil can also calm your body and mind. One common product of eucalyptus essential oil is Vicks Vapor Rub, which you can buy in drugstores and pharmacies.

- Peppermint
  Because of peppermint's antibacterial and antiviral properties, it is considered as one of the top essential oils for cough and cold. This herb contains menthol. Menthol is best known for the relief it gives for congestion so it improves your nasal airflow by unclogging your sinuses. It also gives a cooling sensation which soothes your scratchy throat. Most importantly, it

reduces the severity of your cough which gives discomfort.

You may enjoy these peppermint oil benefits in several ways. Have 3-5 drops of peppermint essential oil in a diffuser as it disperses the vaporized soothing scent as it clears your air passage. You can also topically apply 2-3 drops of the oil to the back of your neck and temples, and chest. If you want to create your own vapor rub, try to mix this oil with eucalyptus essential oil for a more satisfying experience. An important note to observe, do not apply near your eyes as it causes irritation.

- Rosemary
  Rosemary contains cineole, the same substance you can find in eucalyptus which reduces the severity and frequency of cough. The compound cineole also help in breaking the mucus and is a remedy for inflammation. This essential oil boosts the immune system because of its antimicrobial and antioxidant properties. Rosemary also relaxes the muscles in the trachea giving you a respiratory relief.

  For topical application, have 5 drops of rosemary essential oil and directly apply to your chest. Inhalation process is pretty common too so you can just simply inhale a diluted rosemary oil for a faster relief.

For best results, try combining this oil with either peppermint or eucalyptus essential oil. In a recent research, a mixture of these oils helped patients with their cold, cough, and sore throat through inhalation process. Just do it 5 times a day for a few minutes and wait for the favorable results after at least 3 days.

- Tea Tree
  When essential oils were not yet developed, crushed leaves from tea tree oil were used in treating cough, cold, and congestion. Tea tree has many uses and luckily it can also be used as an essential oil for cough and cold. It is best recognized due to its antibacterial, antiseptic, and antimicrobial properties. It has a vitalizing scent and best works in alleviating congestion resulting from cold. It is a powerful protectant against bacteria, which prevents you from having cold and other respiratory symptoms.
  Tea tree essential oil as multipurpose oil comes in many ways to be enjoyed. First, you can have a few drops in a diffuser to alleviate chest congestion. You may also have a generous amount to be directly applied to the back of your neck and temples to relieve headaches and chronic cough. You may also add a few drops of

tea tree oil to a bowl of warm water, soak a towel in the mixture and drape across your chest or head.

- Oregano
Oregano contains a compound called carvacrol. In preliminary research, carvacrol was revealed to have interesting results against cancer cells. It expedited cancer cell death, and at the same time remained nontoxic. But on the later studies, health-promoting benefits of carvacrol when it comes to respiratory symptoms were also proven. Carvacrol can fight off various types of germs as it acts as an antimicrobial agent. It also exhibits antiviral activity, which is very much beneficial in relieving respiratory conditions which may lead to cold and cough.
To enjoy the benefits of oregano essential oil through topical application, rub 2-3 drops of oil mixed with a carrier oil like coconut oil and directly apply to your chest, back, or bottoms of your feet. If you feel symptoms or bacterial conditions which may lead to cough, add a drop or two to a glass of warm water and drink twice daily. However, it was suggested that internal usage of oregano essential oil must be maximized for two week.

The quest for developing natural treatment for different illnesses and ailments never stopped. And since change is constant, our adaptability to external conditions must be stronger. I am referring to our body's adaptability to changes in the weather conditions, to somehow avoid sickness. But as everyone would say, cough and cold is inevitable and might really attack you sometimes of the year. If you catch one, try these essential oils for cough mentioned above. They are easy to use and cause minimal side effects. And since prevention is better than cure, just take your daily vitamins.

The Blending Process

These EOs are categorized by aromas, and EOs from the same group usually blend fantastically together.

- Floral – Lavender, Geranium, Jasmine
- Woodsy – Pine, Cedarwood
- Earthy – Vetiver, Patchouli
- Herbaceous – Marjoram, Rosemary, Basil
- Minty – Peppermint, Spearmint, Wintergreen
- Medicinal – Eucalyptus, Frankincense, Melaleuca
- Spicy – Pepper, Clove, Cinnamon
- Oriental – Ginger, Patchouli
- Citrus – Wild Orange, Lemon, Lime

Select oils that will give you with the health benefits you are looking to remedy. For increased energy choose: Grapefruit, Lemon, Orange, or Citrus. For Calming and Relaxation choose: Lavender, Cedarwood, or Chamomile. You are encouraged to experiment and play with your oils to see which blends work for you.

TIPS:

- Combine Floral EOs with Woodsy, Spicy and Citrus aromas
- Minty EOs with Woodsy, Earthy, Herbaceous and Citrus aromas
- Earthy EOs with Woodsy and Minty aromas
- Citrus EOs with Floral, Woodsy, Minty, Spicy and Oriental aromas

Diffuse

Diffusing Essential Oils is the safest
method to enjoy Essential Oils
without the risk of an allergic reaction.

Diffusing Essential Oils
Some Tidbits You Need To Know

Our sense of smell is one of our most powerful senses, and as you have noticed in your own experience that some scents affect your more positively in your minds than others. The body contains over 1,000 receptors for smell—way more receptors than for any of our other senses.

Diffusion Essential Oils means the process vaporizes oils into the air by releasing tiny amounts into the air. Inhalation is totally safe and is super low risk. Chances of any EO rising to dangerous levels while diffusion is slim to none.

Diffusing Essential Oils around newborns, babies, young children, pregnant or nursing women, and pets should be done with caution. Read up on safety.

It is advisable that Diffusing Essential Oils for only about 15-30 minutes at a time to be most effective. NEVER leave your diffuser on overnight. Make sure your diffuser is filled with the right amount of water and you understand the operating directions.

While diffusing essential oils, be sure that your space has great ventilation. Crack a window open if the scent becomes strong.

Never add Carrier Oils to your diffuser. This may cause your diffuser to malfunction. Clean your diffuser at least 3 times a week with warm water and natural soap to ensure the diffuser is well maintained and bacteria and mold does not accumulate.

Diffusing Essential Oils Basic Guidelines

Just a few things you need to know and prepare before getting started Diffusing Essential Oils.

Things you need:
Ultrasonic Oil Diffuser
Essential Oils
Water

Just follow the number of drops in the recipe, drop on to an oil diffuser and fill the rest with water.

All diffusers are different and will have its own water minimum and maximum level. Read the diffuser instruction before use.

Ideally, it is best to diffuse for 15-30 minutes and turn off the diffuser. The effect should be good for at least 2-3 hours. Turn your diffuser back on after 3 hours to reinforce oil diffusing effects.

It is not advisable to use EO in humidifiers.

These are not made to release EOS

Diffuser Recipes

Here's a thought for you:

You may be wondering how aroma can simply eliminate symptoms. There's a simple answer to this : Aroma is simply a by-product of diffusing. It's the added benefit but in reality the real benefit comes from the air we breathe and how the body easily absorbs the essential oils released into the air. It works 2 ways, not only does it improve the air quality you breath by disinfecting and eliminating pollutants it also allows your glands to absorb the healing elements of the EOs released in the air molecules,

So here are a few recipes that can help you manage symptoms and actual issues regarding the matter :

2 Drops Clove
2 Drops Lemon
2 Drops Cinnamon
2 Drops Eucalyptus
2 Drops Rosemary

----

3 Drops Rosemary
2 Drops Eucalyptus
2 Drops Peppermint
1 Drops Cypress
1 Drops Lemon

----

2 Drops Lemon
1 Drops Lime
2 Drops Peppermint

1 Drops Rosemary
2 Drops Eucalyptus
1 Drops Clove

----

3 Drops RC
3 Drops Lemon
3 Drops Purification

----

2 Drops Eucalyptus
1 Drops Peppermint
3 Drops Frankincense

----

4 Drops Thieves
3 Drops Eucalyptus Radiata
3 Drops Lavender

----

1 Drop Lemon
1 Drop Eucalyptus
2 Drops Peppermint
1 Drop Rosemary

----

1 Drop Rosemary
2 Drops Eucalyptus
2 Drops Lime
1 Drop Peppermint
1 Drops Frankincense

----

2 Drops Frankincense
2 Drops Orange
1 Drop Eucalyptus

----

2 Drops Oregano
2 Drops Rosemary
2 Drops Peppermint
2 Drops Eucalyptus
----

3 Drops Eucalyptus
2 Drops Lavender
2 Drop Peppermint

----

3 Drops Eucalyptus
3 Drops Tea Tree
----

4 Drops Eucalyptus
2 Drops Myrrh
4 Drops Cedarwood

Roll

Essential Oil Roller Bottles is the easiest method to enjoy Essential Oils Anywhere and Whenever.

Blending Essential Oils in a Roller Bottle
Some Tidbits You Need To Know

Essential Oils are usually super concentrated and too hard to measure how much to actually put straight from the bottle.

Roller bottles are a way that you are able to create blends ready to use with the right dilution. It allows your EO to last longer.

It also makes it easier to apply exactly where you want to target without getting it all over the place.

It is handy and easy to carry in your purse, ready to use at any time you want to.

I like to apply EOs at the bottom of the feet for many reasons. Our feet have bigger pores than any other skin in our bodies. this means that they are able to suck in the therapeutic compounds in our blend into the bloodstream faster than any other parts of the body. Imagine comparing a normal straw to an oversized straw and how much more you can suck in with the latter. This is how the soles of our feet is compared to the rest of the skin in our bodies.

The skin on our feet is also less sensitive and is designed to withstand some abuse. The risk of having an irritation from EOS is less likely to happen when applied on the feet.

The feet don't have the glands that act as a barrier. Sebaceous glands are glands in our skin that produces an oily substance called Sebum, for the purpose of lubricating and waterproofing the skin. Since this is oil and if you put oil on top of oil, it can act as a barrier or it may slow down penetration.

The feet and palms of our hands are the only skin that don't have these, so it is ideal to apply Essential Oils to the feet for maximum penetration.

Now, it would be hard to apply oils directly and very messy, right? Roller bottles make it super easy and convenient to roll the EOs at the bottom of our feet.

Carrier Oils Info

Carrier oils are vegetable-based oils with their own healing properties that dilute essential oils used to help carry the EOs into the skin.

Essential oils are highly concentrated and could evaporate very quickly. The carrier oil is mixed with the essential oil so it could penetrate the skin before it actually evaporates. Although EOs are oils, it is actually not that oily. When mixed with a carrier oil, it allows you to have more of the essential oil into your skin without wasting EOS to evaporate, making the healing properties of the EO strong and more effective.

There are also Essential oils that are too strong to apply directly to the skin and may cause damage, so it is important to dilute them with a carrier oil.

Never add Carrier Oils to your diffuser. This may cause your diffuser to malfunction. Clean your diffuser at least 3 times a week with warm water and natural soap to ensure the diffuser is well maintained and bacteria and mold does not accumulate.

Carrier Oils

There are a lot of different carrier oils that you can use with EOs to dilute them in a roller bottle.

To name a few :

Almond Oil - moisturizing and stays liquid at room temperature. Do not use if you are allergic to nuts.

Apricot Kernel Oil - moisturizing and suitable for sensitive skin or kids. It is super gentle on the skin.

Avocado Oil - moisturizing and suitable for sensitive and damaged skin. Perfect for skin problems.Can be mixed with other carrier oils

Castor Oil - with antibacterial, antiviral and antifungal properties, use topically to eliminate pain and relieve skin irritation.

Coconut Oil - its antibacterial, antiviral and antifungal properties it is the best and most versatile for skin care. The skin absorbs this very quickly. It solidifies in room temp and may still have a slight coconut oil aroma in it - but you can get fractionated coconut oil to eliminate the 2 challenges above.

Grapeseed Oil - not just for cooking but also great for topical application on the skin.

Jojoba Oil - one of my faves for skin care blends. This oil is the closest to our natural oil our skin produces to it is absorbed easily without being oily. Also amazing for massage oil blends.

Olive Oil - this is the oil for herb type oils. mostly used for cooking but can also be applied to the skin but would need to be blended with a carrier oil that is mild and absorb well with the skin.

Rosehip Seed Oil - super good for deep moisturizing or skin irritations. This oil has a high content of antioxidants and helps remedy dry, scarred and wounded skin.

Recommended Roller Bottle Dilution Guide

RECOMMENDED ROLL-ON BOTTLE DILUTION AMOUNTS

5 ml (1/6 oz.) Roll-on Bottle = ~100 drops (1tsp.)
10 ml (1/3 oz.) Roll-on Bottle = ~200 drops (2 tsp.)
30 ml. (1 oz.) Roll-on Bottle = ~600 drops (6 tsp.)

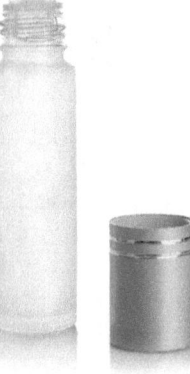

Roll-on Size	5 ml	10 ml	30 ml	Add EO drops to roll-on, then fill with carrier oil.	
Essential Oil Drops	1	2	6	1%	Dilution Percentage
	2	4	12	2%	
	3	6	18	3%	
	5	10	30	5%	
	10	20	60	10%	
	20	40	120	20%	
	25	50	150	25%	
	50	100	300	50%	

General Guidelines:
Birth to 12 months = .3-.5% dilution
1-5 years = 1.5-3% dilution
6-11 years = 1.5-5% dilution
12-17 years = 1.5-20% dilution
18 years and older = 1.5% dilution-Neat (no dilution)
Elderly or Sensitive Skin = 1-3% dilution
Daily Use = 2-5% dilution
Short Term Use = 10-25% dilution
Local Skin or Systemic Issues = 50% dilution-Neat

These are general guidelines suggestions--not absolute rules--based on traditional aromatheraphy practice.
(Kurt Schnaubelt PhD, Valerie Worwood, Robert Tisserand)

Dilution Basics:

How much you dilute your EO depends on different factors such as weight, sensitivity, health conditions, EOs that are blended in or how long that blend has been used for. There is never an absolute dilution rule, it is you who knows about your level and tolerance. I feel that it is best to start with a higher dilution percentage and increase EO drops over time.

To make sure your EO is safe, make sure that the oils you use are therapeutic grade and do your research on the source and extraction methods used to produce the oils.

Roller Bottle Blending Order

I normally just start with dropping the drops of oil into the **10mL roller bottle**, then adding the carrier oil up until the shoulder of the bottle. Capping the bottle off with the roller and the bottle cap. Instead of shaking the bottle, i like to roll the bottle between my palms first for a minute or 2 for blending, then finishing it off with a few shakes.

NOTE: All recipes in this book is for a 10mL Roller Bottle. If you have a bigger or smaller roller bottle, adjust the number of EO drops based on the size of your bottle.

Roller Bottle Recipes

5 drops Onguard
5 drops Oregano
5 drops Lemon
----

10 drops Respiratory Blend
6 drops Lime
----

5 drops Eucalyptus
3 drops Frankincense
2 drops Lemon
----

8 drops Breathe
5 drops Lime
----

6 drops Respiratory Blend
4 drops Eucalyptus
3 drops Frankincense
----

4 drops Lemon
4 drops Peppermint
2 drops Frankincense
----

6 drops RC
4 drops Lemon
4 drops Purification
2 drops Thyme
----

3 drops Lemon
3 drops Clove
3 drops Eucalyptus
3 drops Rosemary

----

4 drops Oregano
6 drops Lemon
5 drops On Guard
5 drops Melaleuca

----

4 drops Frankincense
4 drops Lemon
4 drops Melaleuca Tea Tree
4 drops Protective Blend

----

2 drops Oregano
2 drops Melaleuca
2 drops Lemon
2 drops Frankincense
2 drops Cinnamon

----

3 drops Orange
3 drops Lemon
3 drops Thieves
3 drops Frankincense

----

4 drops Thieves
4 drops Purification
4 drops Oregano
----

8 drops Respiratory Blend
5 drops Eucalyptus
4 drops Frankincense
----

6 drop Cardamom
6 drop Frankincense
----

2 drops Oregano
2 drops Tea Tree
2 drops Lemon
2 drops Frankincense
2 drops Cinnamon
----

4 drops Peppermint
2 drops Eucalyptus
2 drops Lemon
2 drops Rosemary
----

2 drops Lemon
6 drops Lavender
2 drops Peppermint
----

4 drops Peace & Calming
3 drops Lavender

3 drops Frankincense

Bonus Recipes

Geranium Lotion

½ cup Shea Butter
6-7 drops Sea Buckthorn Oil
6-7 drops Rosehip Seed Oil
6-7 drops Geranium Oil
1 teaspoon Avocado Oil

Peppermint Moisturizer

3 tablespoons Sweet Almond Oil
1 tablespoon Avocado Oil
3 teaspoons Beeswax
2 drops Lavender Essential Oil
2 tablespoons Mineral Water
1 drop Peppermint Essential Oil

Rose Soap

⅓ cup castile soap
⅓ cup raw honey
⅓ cup olive oil
30-60 drops essential oils (use a blend of oils
such as sweet orange, vanilla, and lavender)

Vanilla Body Spray

1 cup Distilled Water
2 tablespoons Vegetable Glycerin
1 drop of your favorite essential oil

Vanilla Extract Scrub

¼ cup Olive Oil
1 teaspoon Pure Vanilla Extract
1 cup Brown Turbinado Sugar
15 drops Peppermint Essential Oil
½ cup Used Coffee Grounds from a Freshly
Brewed Pot

Rose Cleansing Solution

¼ cup Aloe Vera gel
1 teaspoon of carrier oil
1 teaspoon Glycerin
5 drops Rosemary

Patchouli

1 tsp Carrier Oil (argan, coconut, sesame,
sweet almond, jojoba, grapeseed,
macadamia)
2 drops Chamomile
2 drops Palmarosa
1 drop Patchouli

Inhale

Essential Oil Inhalers are the most convenient way to enjoy Essential Oils Anywhere and Whenever.

Essential Oil Inhalers give you quick and easy access to the vast therapeutic benefits of essential oils.

Blending Essential Oils in an Inhaler
Some Tidbits You Need To Know

EO Inhalers or aroma sticks are compact tubes, with a cotton wick inside and a protective cover, to lock the aroma within.

Your preferred blend of essential oils is absorbed by the cotton wick, and safely enclosed in a tube that fits inside of the cover. The cover is easily removed for access to the tube to breathe in the aroma. Usually lasts about 3 months, depending on the oil blend used.

I absolutely love these because they encourage me to take a moment during super stressful moments, and just breathe.

It is in times of stress when our breathing patterns often change and taking deep breaths promote a feeling of calm and inner peace. Breath work combined with visualization plus a relaxing inhaler, can offer relief to symptoms of stress and help your body to come back to the state of homeostasis.

Aroma Sticks can be carried in your tiny purse, even compact enough to fit in your pocket. You can enjoy your favorite EOs anywhere and you can use them with discretion.

I love diffusing, and do all the time but not everyone in my space may enjoy the scents I enjoy or they may not benefit from the therapeutic benefits of the EOs I am diffusing - so the inhaler is one way to not only enjoy my choice of blends but to keep in personal not affecting everyone else around me.

Inhalers not only benefits me but also keep those around me safe in case the oils I want to blend may pose a risk to those around me who may have a health issue not advised to be exposed to my choice EOs/

When making Aroma Sticks, You may use your chosen EOs at 100% Concentration.

Inhaler Basic Guidelines

Breathe in slow and deep to absorb the EO molecules directly into your olfactory system.

Inhalers are super easy to use. You just remove the cap and inhale from the inhaler tube, count 1 to 5 slowly as you inhale. The EO molecules get drawn into our bloodstream through our nasal cavity and gets delivered throughout our entire body.

Simple to use, easy to cary, portable and compact. You never have to be without your favorite blends, ever.

Inhaler Blending Basics

Inhalers are super easy and simple to make.

All you need is an inhaler set which consist of the following:

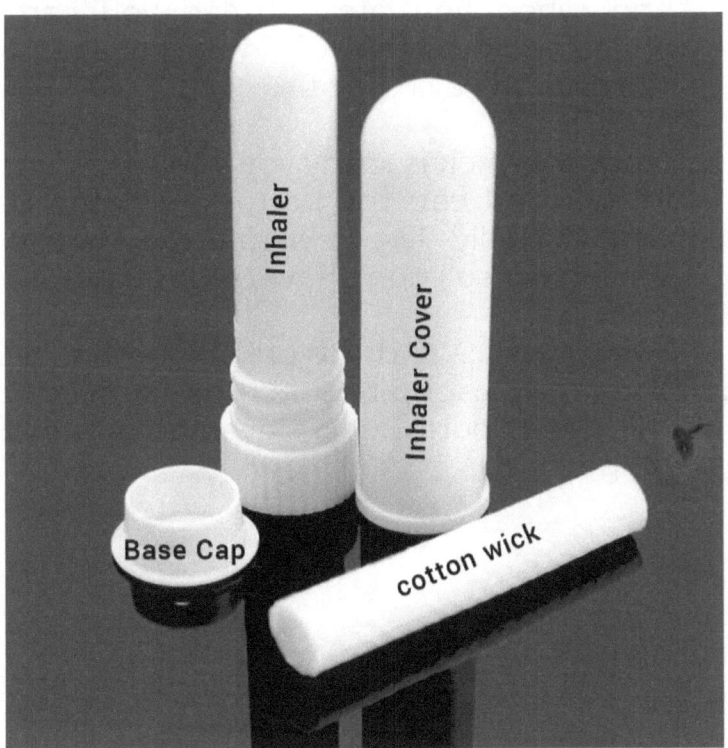

Inhaler, Inhaler Cover, Base Cap and Cotton Wick.

You will need your Essential Oils.

I like to use a pipette for precision and a small petri dish so I can see the oil.

Blending is super easy, just combine the drops and swirl it around in the petri dish and when you are satisfied you can go ahead and drop the cotton wick to absorb all the oil in the dish.

Once the wick is ready you can drop it in the inhaler and cap the bottom with the Base Cap. I usually like to secure the cover with the inhaler so I don't have to do it later.

I usually us 15-20 drops of EO total in a recipe and it can last up to 3 months. Some recipes will need more but on average it is in this range.

Inhaler Recipes

3 drops Oregano
3 drops Tea Tree
3 drops Lemon
3 drops Frankincense
3 drops Cinnamon Leaf

----

5 drops Peppermint
5 drops Eucalyptus
3 drops Lavender
3 drops Lemon
3 drops Rosemary

----

6 drops Rosemary
8 drops Peppermint
6 drops Eucalyptus

----

8 drops Rosemary
5 drops Thyme
2 drops Peppermint

----

12 drops Eucalyptus
8 drops Lavender

----

5 drops of Peppermint

5 drops of Eucalyptus
2 drops of Lavender
2 drops of Lemon
2 drops of Rosemary

----

5 drops of Eucalyptus
5 drops of Siberian Fir
5 drops of Peppermint

----

9 drops Rosemary
3 drop Thyme
3 drop Peppermint
----

7 drops of Pine or Cedarwood
7 drops of Lavender
4 drops of Eucalyptus
1 drop of Lemon
----

8 drops of Rosemary
8 drops of Peppermint
6 drops of Eucalyptus
----

10 drops of Rosemary
4 drops of Thyme
2 drops of Peppermint
----

6 drops of Pine or Rosemary
6 drops of Peppermint
4 drops of Eucalyptus

----

9 drops of Rosemary
3 drops of Thyme
3 drops of Peppermint

----

6 drops of Spruce
4 drops of Eucalyptus
3 drops of Lemon
2 drops of Lime

----

5 drops of Frankincense
6 drops of Lavender
4 drops of Wild Orange

----

6 drops of Eucalyptus
3 drops of Roman Chamomile
6 drops of Frankincense

----

4 drops of Cedarwood
6 drops of Roman Chamomile
10 drops of Frankincense

----

8 drops of Thieves
4 drops of Frankincense
4 drops of Lemon

----

5 drops of Lemon
5 drops of Lavender
5 drops of Peppermint

----

3 drops of Oregano
3 drops of Tea Tree
3 drops of Lemon
3 drops of Frankincense
3 drops of Cinnamon

----

9 drops of Hyssop
5 drops of Black Spruce
3 drops of Lavender
1 drop of Peppermint

----

3 drops of Black Spruce
6 drops of Lavender
6 drops of Scotch Pine
3 drops of Spearmint

XX

Book Ordering

To order your copy / copies of

Essential Oils
for Colds

please visit: **EOrecipes.net**

You can also check out other titles
available.

Bulk Pricing and
Affiliate Programs Available